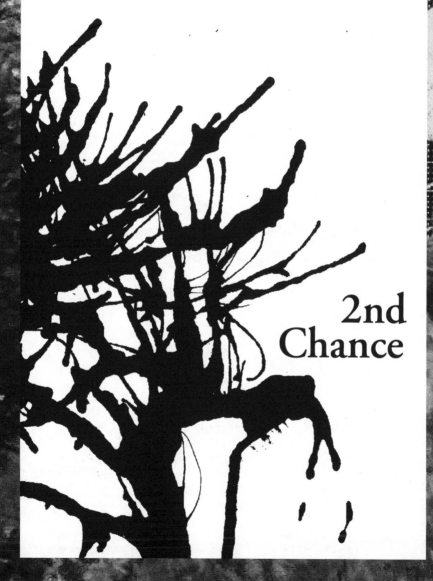

2nd
Chance

New Issues Poetry & Prose

Editor	Nancy Eimers
Managing Editor	Kimberly Kolbe
Copy Editor	Abigail Goodhart
Assistant Editor	Abigail Goodhart

New Issues Poetry & Prose
The College of Arts and Sciences
Western Michigan University
Kalamazoo, MI 49008

First Edition, 2020.

ISBN-13   978-1-936970-67-4 (paperbound)

Library of Congress Cataloging-in-Publication Data:
Becker, Daniel M.
2nd Chance/Daniel M. Becker
Library of Congress Control Number: 2020938683

Art Director	Nick Kuder
Designer	Corby Deford
Production Manager	Paul Sizer
	The Design Center, Frostic School of Art
	College of Fine Arts
	Western Michigan University
Printing:	McNaughton & Gunn, Inc.

2nd Chance

Daniel M. Becker

New Issues Press

WESTERN MICHIGAN UNIVERSITY

For Linn

Contents

Acknowledgements

Ars Medica: "Before Flu Season"

Forklift: Ohio: "Reading Middlebrow Cosmology"

Hektoen International: "Advance Directives"

JAMA (Journal of the American Medical Association): "Home Visit"
   "After Life and In Between," "In Memoriam," and "Twilight"

Journal of General Internal Medicine: "Physic for Poets"

Mudlark: "Goals of Care"

Nimrod: "In the Office of the Balance Center Director,"
   "Bulkheads,"and "Like All Perfect Strangers"

Poet Lore: "Standing in Line at *Pet Forum*"

Pulse: "Swimming with John's Ghost," "Sleep Hygiene,"
   "This Is Not a Drill," "Best Story Teller Award," "Consult,"
   and "At Medical Center Hour"

Rattle: "Joint National Commissions Galore"

Consult

A minute after the tube is out she turns blue and stops moving. Half a minute later she loses her pulse. I learned as a student to feel the difference between the pulse in my fingers and the pulse at the patient's wrist. Or thought I learned. When you listen for a heart to stop you start to hear heart sounds that might not be there. Like waking up at night thinking you heard something then listening to the dark to be sure, not quite convinced either way. Weak sounds, S1 and S2, valves closing. Slow and slower, regular then irregular, then almost nothing…then who knows?

The monitor is off in her room but on at the nursing station. One screen shows every heart in the unit. I don't want to sign the consult note until the line stays flat. *Erratic electrical activity went on for a few minutes* is an understatement.

She'd be gone for most of the screen then come back for a complex or two then go away again. I watch the blip travel left to right then arrive at the edge of the screen then turn a corner out of sight and get lost until out of nowhere it finds itself and comes back from the other side. Several nurses stop what they're doing to watch too. Finally, I discharge her from the monitor.

Among the Deep Listeners in Deep Listening 101

are music majors taking the class for credit
and an auditor on Social Security
who can only hum one note and that's the note he hums.
Overtones find a major chord. Then we march off and find a place to sit
and list the sounds while building castles out of sound.
Listening is the hardest thing a brain does
according to listening psychologists
soliciting grants and donations.
It is now possible to follow sound into the brain
and map its journey up the brainstem and into the attic.
Some sounds turn on all the lights.
Other sounds turn them off.
In one creation myth human ears fly like bats
from one echo to another.
The bats returning to our attic
don't trigger the motion detector in our driveway.
It takes poetic license to claim that motion detectors listen
unless the motion detector is a sleeping dog
who wakes up to announce the UPS truck in the driveway.
Look around, listen up: there are worlds beyond our thresholds.

During the field trip inside the sound free chamber:
those strangers pounding at the door?
Heart beats.

We're Talking about What to Look for When Listening

and the lively discussion about intonation,
whether it counts as verbal or nonverbal,
leaves me scratching my head, in a manner of speaking.

Leaning forward means getting closer, and that's true
in any language, especially true for bad news sinking in.
Eye contact can be too much of a good thing.

Someone taught me to stare at the nose not the eyes
in order to keep a safe distance. That works, but there you are,
a serious conversation, studying every pore on some poor nose.

Someone claims we can teach monkeys to stare, and heads nod,
but I'm not so sure. Dogs yes. Their dark eyes beckon.
The point is that body language should emerge—a rheostat? —

otherwise some nonverbals are too bright, too loud, too taught.
It's hard to know what to dial in, but a pause,
then a figurative hand on the shoulder, a parenthetical hand.

Picture the kind teacher asking that quiet kid,
so quiet it's disquieting, *still with us?*
That's what us quiet kids are here to learn.

What can we learn from all the different ways patients say
I don't know
during memory tests they happen to be failing?

Shrugs, eye contact running on empty,
long slow looks out the window
if we're lucky enough to have a window

that offers something else to think about.
Remember 3 objects:
house, car, cow. While they wander around in the attic

I picture that cow with blue light explaining its back,
the same blue as the mountains standing behind the herd
in my friend's painting of October.

Not our mountains, but October is October.
In every room in every conference there's someone who talks too much,
someone to tune out while talking to yourself

and looking out the window that isn't there and thinking hard
about intonation at the lectern and tone on the page.
You don't need to say the words to hear them and own them.

Tone inflects meaning, except for the Norwegians here—
an international meeting—who inflect the end of every sentence.
As do the French—*n'est-ce pas?*—but with a different scale.

We add meaning as we listen, for instance the dog
that comes, sits, and drools whenever he hears the whistle.
As for what the other senses are trying to tell us:

who's to say what experience is?
When Sappho says
mere air these words, but delicious to hear

might what fizzed for her taste flat to me?
I can't taste those hints of blackberry in the wine,
but if that concept wants to waft up to the brain

where the blackberries are waiting to remind me
how they grew wild along the fence between our field
and what used to be the cow field

shouldn't I try to listen? Who can forget those cows
or how their field ends at the woods crossed by a stream
that leads to a river where we cool off on a hot day?

The dogs like that. In fact, their dark eyes beckon.

In the Office of the Balance Center Director

around the corner from Audiology
on a desk near a model of the inner ear
a dozen paperweights are waiting.

The Director picks one up to make it snow and illustrate
how the brain knows where the head is heading.
From the desktop of her laptop she double-clicks a film clip

of two eyes gazing to the left and ticking like a watch—
clockwise when sitting, counter clockwise when supine—
since disembarking from a cruise across an ocean.

Eyes adjust to lost horizons, but first they need to wander.
Her finger tracks the voyage of the otoliths, calcite crystals,
bone and stone that aren't supposed to float but on occasion do.

On a related subject the 3rd auditory ossicle
in the deep end of the middle ear
is as small as "In God" on a dime, if you've ever read a dime.

Hearing and balance, two sides of one coin,
depend on endolymph in motion to activate the auditory nerve.
Vertigo can be loud as a tunnel or quiet as a cricket,

a *silver cricket* the patient explains.

Joint National Commissions Galore

I like the new cholesterol guidelines
better than the old guidelines: no room for confusion,
like the signs at the edge of a flat world.

But with or without guidelines, arteries harden and narrow,
and somewhere inside each of us
the blood will make a *whoosh whoosh* sound

while getting to where it is going.
In med school *Professor Lub Dub Smith* taught us how
to listen to the *lub dub* sounds

that heart valves make as they close in sequence.
He would stand at the podium and imitate the heart
adding clicks, murmurs, rumbles, gallops, and snaps

according to where the heart was troubled.
We loved him standing up there and sounding
like an exotic male bird showing off for the ladies.

I offer my stethoscope to the patient who *whooshes*,
but either he's not ready for our ears to touch by proxy
or hearing his own clogged artery is too much information.

But a little too close for comfort is how we learn,
that's how we know exactly where to listen.
If one day I look in one ear and out the other

I'll never make that joke again.
I'd issue the standard warning
against going too far with *Q Tips* and leave it at that.

People don't need to know everything, all the details
that don't matter. Why the chloride is high
is like asking why normal is normal and then you need

to go statistic and draw the normal distribution in the air,
taking the audience out there on one tail or the other
of the bell-shaped curve, at which point they take my hand

from whatever horizon it's pointing at and say *it's ok,
it's going to be ok.* Not normal isn't so bad.
Each result on the chem 20 panel has a 5% chance

of being too high or low, and the chance of a normal person
being normal for everything is about 50%, lower than you'd guess.
When I give that lecture the students look out the window

to check if the grass is still growing.
Later in life, they will recount eternity in an hour
and apply that wisdom to their daily yoga practice,

not only apply it but rub it in to achieve a care free finish.
People don't know care free
until an asteroid out of nowhere blots it and the horizon out

then crashes through the ceiling so there's no place to sit
except on the edge of a speck of the big bang.
In that gloomy light what looks like a mixed metaphor

turns out is an elephant hogging the sofa.
Best not to talk too much about something like that,
best to reframe that experience, after all

it was only a small asteroid, maybe just a meteor,
a shooting star, someone's wish wishing to come true.
The doctors say *maybe we can help a little*

and the patient decides *a little chemo* sounds better
than nothing. It's easier to hear what we want to hear,
and not just because of ear wax or the vacuum

that used to be memory or good old reliable denial—
which may be dumb but is not stupid—
but because of Charles Darwin and natural selection.

Counting on happy endings helps us reproduce,
impose sanctions, plan for retirement, trust sun screen,
overcome modesty, fall in love and stay in love

like that lively couple French kissing on the beach
while I was getting a sun burn.
The French also invented the stethoscope. *Whoosh*

you want to hear him whisper in her ear.
Their private joke. *Shush* her private answer.
His cholesterol looks high, sugar and blood pressure too,

the kind of more than chunky more than middle age guy
who falls dead more often than chance would allow.
Is laughter his best medicine?

Not according to the Joint National Commission.
With electronic medical records, it's easy to rank patients
with diabetes and learn the higher numbers are people

who like to thank the staff with home baked cookies.
It's a sweet gesture. Sharing makes them happy.
We let them be happy, but we can't make them,

not that there are guidelines. You can make
an old friend happy just by bumping into him
on the sidewalk. He'll say how happy he is to see you.

Then say it again to make it stick. You smile back.
You stop slouching. You know that feeling when you finally
get around to changing the light bulb in the garage

and can go in there and actually see? That's how light it feels:
two old friends watching the dawn until the indoor pool opens.
Cholesterol doesn't come up,

but staying alive is implied by context. Why else be up early
swimming laps and asking existential questions?
Why does the water feel cold even though it isn't?

Why keep the locker room so cold? Why do goggles
fit perfect one day and leak the next?
Same head, same beady little Kafka eyes that are overdue,

according to the postcard, for a check-up.
There's a moment during that exam
when the reflection of the optic nerve

is visible to its owner, just a glimpse is all you get,
it seeing you seeing it, hardly counts as introspection
but what could be more meta?

Halls of mirrors for one thing. Guidelines for another.
Thousands of randomized patients and after a while
they look so much like you or me that escape is impossible.

While standing in line getting guidelined to death,
while explaining to the nurse your pressure is always high
at the doctor's office, while saying *aah* then saying *aah*

an octave higher, while trying as instructed twice
to *please don't blink the eye drops out*—
staring as hard as you can to be a good patient—

think about how hard it is to outwit a reflex.
They never listen. Think about all those basic circuits
lined up end to end, how they can take us to the moon

and back if only we would let them.
Last night there was a full lunar eclipse,
the kind that looks like cream of tomato soup,

all the sunrises and sunsets on the planet
bent in the moon's direction. But it was raining hard,
cats and dogs, too wet for shadows, and the rain

was an excuse to stay in bed and listen
to three points form a straight line
while heading in different directions.

The night purred as it settled into place.

Reading Middlebrow Cosmology

From nowhere, Quantum the cat leaps on the bed
where I am stuck on Kepler's second law—
the area swept by a planet's orbit

makes me think of windshield wipers.
I have forgotten more geometry
than most people learn.

There's a cat pinned to my chest.
The universe shrinks to the size of the closest chest,
mine at the moment, and unraveling,

but what's a moment in the life of a sweater,
dark blue and knitted, like the sky.
Cosmology because we're between moons,

stars tapping on the tin roof,
and gravity, the weakest force, is in the news again.
Cosmology because this morning

I sat and stood and sat and stood in synagogue
where I have forgotten more Hebrew
than most people learn, and to pass the time

I found something to read in English,
reading past Creation to the people,
tracing begats and admonition all the way to Noah.

Ask me the size of the Ark in cubits.
A cubit is the length of someone's forearm,
more unbidden knowledge, but don't ask me in a week.

Think of heaven as the night and night as a sponge
soaked with dark matter. To learn the age of the universe
work back from its edge, except it's a sphere

with four dimensions and perhaps not even peerless.
Look around and ask like Leibniz why something
rather than nothing. First the big bang, now the cat purrs,

and in the space-time continuum
I sit, globe spinning in my lap,
taking nothing and everything for granted.

I grew up here, under my finger, by the ocean,
and this is my life now, by the mountains.
The daily planet and the next, tunnels of time,

the tunnel of love, light that bends in homage
to the weight of darkness outside our darkness.

Home Visit

We follow a blue Ford tractor pulling a wagon
and moving slowly, scattering straw like exhaust,
Southside Virginia in July, still haying season,
so hot the haze shimmies on the asphalt,
June bugs strafe the windshield,
the afternoon breeze a warm sponge.
The nurse is the guide, telling me
how to greet other drivers,
lift two fingers from the steering wheel,
only two, show some restraint;
where to park—watch out for the dog, stretching a yawn,
scored ribs settling on a minor chord;
who's who as we edge through the home
front porch to back, generations un-gapped,
no work, no school, no a/c. Fans whir,
TV promises a better life.
We reach the kitchen, and in the pantry
an old woman with electric hair
and petrified eyes hums a gospel.
She looks straight through us.
She's expecting Jesus, sweet Jesus.

Twilight

He lights a cigarette and explains
that if it was safe to smoke in the engine room
of a World War II destroyer
then it is safe to smoke near his oxygen
flowing two liters every minute.
When my two years of pre-med chemistry
suggest his hot air chemistry's at sea,
he quotes Alexander Pope
on how a little knowledge is dangerous.
While he catches his breath, I quote Pope
on bias and pride. Then he quotes Pope
on error and forgiveness. After we've run out of Pope
but still on the subject of safety, he shows me the gun
in the bedside table drawer, there in easy reach,
safety on, self-defense he wants me to know.
I get to see the gun at every visit.
What's a bed doing in a sitting room?
This is his favorite subject we've agreed
to disagree on. *Just lying there* I answer.
I push the button that changes lying to sitting.
He pushes the button that lets him sit where he prefers.
He pours the brandy he's so proud of.
Once a month we have this conversation,
and once a month he doesn't drink alone.

The Best Story Teller Award

At the clinic retreat everyone gets a prize,
and the *Best Story Teller* reminds us of those times
a man goes on a journey. But this man is Dr. William Osler—

the doctors' doctor, the professors' professor—
and he's crossing the Delaware to Camden where Walt Whitman—
the great American poet, the poet's poet—

endures fame and poor health.
Every case is supposed to be interesting, but Whitman,
according to Osler, suffered only from what his age could explain

plus or minus the usual wear and tear, the side effects and worries,
the incidentals that let doctors hedge their bets.
Chance, then as now, regressed to the mean.

A stroke, then as now, was what it is.
Tuberculosis, then as now, was in the air.
Whitman died from or with tuberculosis.

Osler lived with prosector's warts from more than one
of the hundreds of TB-ridden autopsies
his curiosity insisted on.

When Whitman says *the poet drags the dead out of their coffins
and stands them on their feet,*
the story then wants to see them walk,

and in a tale about a man who crosses a river
listeners feel the breeze and the motion
while doctors recall that case of disembarkation vertigo

and how easy it is for life to be uneasy.
Osler, between two shores, puzzles over Whitman's *Leaves of Grass.*
Whitman, between revisions, puzzles over *Leaves of Grass.*

The housekeeper's cat can't resist the poet's great lap.
The ferry fights the current. At least one passenger is queasy
while the story moves to the next generation of doctors and poets.

When Dr. William Carlos Williams lived in Philadelphia,
he studied Osler and Whitman and where to draw the line
between uncertainty and mystery

and how to make a line of poetry speak for everyone
while the poet earns a living as a doctor.
In the story of the stranger coming to clinic,

our new patients will wait months for 40 minutes.

Physic for Poets

We teach poetry writing to seniors and last night
the subject was food, as in what does your favorite taste like?
There are two Lucys, and my Lucy shakes her head:
fried chicken tastes like chicken.
So much depends on the taste of chicken.

The day before I drove to Free Union to visit a centenarian
who hasn't said a word in years but clicks when she swallows
and trusts her niece with a spoon.
They're snuggled up to the mountains, mountains from every porch.
We talk about diet and dosing and language versus clicks.
I ask about bears because out here everyone has had a bear on the porch.
We are looking at trees, each tied to a sleeping dog,
and the niece says *I was in the driveway and had that feeling*
something was watching me, you know that feeling?
I love that feeling. In others. I listen hard.
The shade is blue and closing in. I should know what time it is.
I'm waiting for the bear, waiting for the niece to turn,
but first she puts her groceries down,
bread and milk, seedless rye and 2%,
then slowly, and there, eye to eye:
the neighbor's emu jumped the fence.
Neck as long as its vowels.
Tastes like chicken.

Once, too, a bear, a cub treed by the dogs.
I type up Lucy's poems. Last week was chicks
and how they turn yellow and grow up to get fried.
She asks *Danny? Is that your name, Danny?*
I thought it was Bobby. Then Alice leans close and says
you stole my teacher. Her poem is popcorn.

Goals of Care

During a bedside conversation
about slippery slopes and failure to thrive
we consider every option,

whatever it takes to get him home
to the second-floor bed where he belongs.
It may take piano movers.

I know their piano teacher.
I know their piano teacher's teacher.
They're still learning what kind of perfect

practice can accomplish.
In my medical opinion a harpsicord, no pedals,
would be easier for high mileage knees and ankles.

I've never played one, but a college roommate
played *Dance of the Marionettes*—
the theme song to *Alfred Hitchcock Presents*—

on a harpsichord he built from a kit.
So what? their faces ask.
So, there's a lot more to talk about:

avoidance versus denial, dignity versus gravitas,
gravity versus pressure sores,
hospital beds versus recliners,

sponge baths versus slipping and falling in the shower,
indwelling versus *in and out* catheterization,
hospice versus home health, PT versus OT

versus lying around hoping for the best,
the clinical utility of faith in a cozy hereafter
versus nothing—not even a vacuum

with good Ouija board reception.
The first hospices were for bodies that acted dead,
but in those days you waited a few days

to be sure not to bury the living,
which brings us to the 21st century ICU
and modern versions of perpetuity

and families who choose that
and doctors and nurses who judge that.
We cross ICU off the list.

After pianos, harpsichords, and advance directives
but getting back to Hitchcock:
you never know when he or someone like him

will insist on entering the conversation.
After all, he was famous for his cameos.
At clinic the other day I was explaining vertigo

to the victim of a rear end collision
and the husband, spiraling his finger, asks
like the movie? Exactly I spiraled back.

Life might imitate art, and we might smile
when the unexpected matches the unexpected,
we might be grateful for the chance to change the subject,

but often, and sadly, after pianos, harpsichords,
advance directives, and elephants in the living room,
there's durable medical equipment

still waiting for third party approval, waiting forever
if that's what it takes. Just last week I was talking to
the shipping clerk at the catheter supply warehouse,

not really talking, begging. Not really begging,
preaching about doing the right thing on a Friday afternoon,
a holiday three-day weekend,

a long time for a bladder not to empty.
Someone might have mentioned something
about Dante's *Inferno* and poetic justice.

It is possible to do the right thing
and it doesn't help to get all holy
or complain about the music when they put you on hold—

that wasn't just a flight of fancy, that was Liberace—
or worry too much about reusing a catheter
after giving it the soft-boiled egg treatment.

Maybe I'm sharing too much?
We're sharing the window seat.
We're in those yellow anti-MRSA gowns

so we talk about normal bacterial skin flora
and how it changes for the worse
with repeated hospitalization,

which brings us to the Book of Job
and whether Job's boils were the Biblical version
of the particular community MRSA that festers.

We don't need the Bible to know that life's tests
aren't supposed to be fair.
The thing about unfairness is how unrelenting it is,

like a stiff prostate—the root cause of a stiff bladder
and recurrent urosepsis, except we call it sepsis of urinary origin
because of a Medicare loophole.

The thing about human knowledge is
how after the fact it is, like a broken hip
after a ground-level fall while trying one step at a time

up the 16 steps to the bedroom.
Sooner or later these conversations lead to
who else can help at home: friends, dear friends,

kids, grandkids, strangers rented by the hour,
and, rather than just sitting there watching someone napping
which good books to read at the bedside?

Which music to listen to? Something *andante*,
but not, I gather, *Dance of the Marionettes*.
So there we are, draped in yellow, adjusting the shades

so the sun stops interrupting, bragging about our kids,
awarding the *grandson of the year* award,
trying not to worry too much about what happens next,

trying to be practical, to make lists, to revise lists,
to face facts, to craft solutions, to test solutions,
to laugh off a little more than necessary,

and we shouldn't hug, because of the germs,
but we do.

Before Flu Season

It's a bunionette not a bunion,
not a rock or shell or glass bead
wedged between the base of the fifth toe
and the inside of her slipper.
A sharp little knife, a #10 blade,
pares away the keratin.
With her heel in the palm of my hand,
we talk about callus and the glory days
of soft skin and cotillions that defied gravity.
I tell her the children's story of the little mouse
who went to visit his mother
and on the way wore out two sets of wheels, a pair of shoes,
both feet. *What nice new feet you have* his mother says
as mothers will.
The patient doesn't get it.
It's one of those stories where
you had to be there, one of those stories
where money buys anything and then a happy ending.
Flecks of dead skin fly off.
The big pieces click on the tile
as we whittle away our time together.
We move from convex to concave,
from literal to rhetorical.
What's the difference between a hole
and half a hole? Is flu vax
safe as well as effective?
This is easy. This is fun.
This is maybe a little weird.
I remember my mother's feet.

Security Questions

Now that death certificates are filled out online
there's one more username
and set of security questions to answer

when trying to reset a password that got misbegotten
or typo'd once too often to be trusted.
What was your favorite movie as a child?

When *Decedent Affairs* asks *"Ghostbusters?"*
what he means is *what possessed you?*
He also knows the name of my senior prom date.

Life can be cuter than fiction. Or too cute.
The online death registry wants me to click on the open coffin icon.
When my father and I went to shop for my mother's coffin

I was young enough that buying beer felt grown-up.
The salesman took us straight to the mahogany aisle.
Veneer was an option.

A patient of mine built the dream house with his own hands
and when the time came he built the solid dream coffin.
His wife was trying to slip away quietly

while he hammered in the morning, hammered in the evening.
He needed to be ready, and when it got close to backhoe time
he asked me if she'd mind listening to her grave clatter up the hillside.

He already knew that noise did not bother her.
She already knew what was coming
and stayed busy quilting the quilt they wrapped her in.

Another husband explains there are worse things in life than dying.
But why did she die? he needed to know, as did the state.
The biology, not the theology.

That conversation moved from spark plugs to brain stems
to heart beats to vital statistics and from there to public health,
epidemics and their vectors, how many legs a flea has,

plague, and the *not dead yet* scene from another favorite movie as a kid.
Both of us smile—a time to weep, a time to laugh,
a time to avoid thinking too hard.

You don't need to be a thanatologist or a sad clown
to know that tragedy is failed comedy.
One mid-summer night the phone rings.

Two wives on the line. One not-on-call-husband
outside sealing the pine deck and feeding the bugs
and the other husband cold and stiff in bed.

Hold on my wife says.
Why him why now what next the new widow laments.
God-dammit she scolds the volume control on the speaker phone.

I know how that feels.
Flatline. Long gone the Rescue Squad reports.
Was this man really your patient? the sheriff investigates.

Really? I ask the moths worshipping the light bulb.
I'm leaning on the brush I'd been mindfully pushing
and saving my mindful sigh in case the widow's doorbell rings

to announce the pizza guy at the wrong door.
The sealant smells water proof but not light proof.
Bad timing for product remorse. I sit down.

My wife sits next to me.
Our shoulders lean in and take up the slack.
After I call the Funeral Home I finish sealing the deck

I should have been staining.
We end up replacing pressure treated pine with mahogany,
but even mahogany will warp without concrete footings

and buttressed joists, like cathedrals, or shoulders.
That deck is my favorite place to be despite the no-see-ums in the summer.
I'm their favorite customer.

Decedent Affairs has a screened in porch
where after a long day of keeping and resetting secrets
he can log off and glow in the dark until it's time for supper.

After Life and In Between

A child has died but is brought back
and remembers floating near the ceiling

looking down at the doctor who is now on the air
sharing the proto-ghost's point of view

with a radio audience, except it's called a near death.
The defibrillator didn't want to work.

The music of spheres whistled like a train.
The proverbial tunnel of light was actually a noodle.

There were clouds too, and baby clouds.
Everyone was nice, especially God.

The doctor chuckles and recalls a couple hundred kids
under ice or in the river long enough to be blue,

stiff, flat-line, gone, ready at last to receive
all benefit of doubt. In the car at 50 miles per hour

and late again for your morning, you hope
when the time comes you can drown first

then reappear beneath those generous hands.
That first breath would taste like lightning.

What I Like about Gout

Before the Godzillionaires hatched
life wasn't half bad
except that occasional catastrophe

the law of averages adjusted for.
The weight of the world hadn't gained all that weight.
Everyone's back didn't have a story.

If on a scale of 1 to 10, and 1 is a weightless day
up there on the international space station
enjoying a nice view of a sleeping universe,

and 10 is down here on a half-baked double-booked planet
where it's still only Monday and harder than it should be
to find the consent form that lets rehab confirm or deny

someone was but is no longer and can't be their patient
unless she happens to get pregnant—
a loophole in the pay as you go standard of care's business plan—

then a period that's two weeks late
is what's left of hope on an average day
in bad choice times at last chance clinic

where we're prisoners of our faxes.
It's hard to know where craving ends and withdrawing begins
I point out to the student who points out

the send button on the fax machine.
My craving is that *get me a social worker and make it quick*
blend of righteousness and sorrow

that's never someone else's problem.
The next 10 flashes hello with 10 fingers,
answering a question that hadn't been asked.

What's new is getting his life back on track
after a 90-day detour for *nothing too egregious*
on a license he forgot was suspended.

In the Olympics, no one gets a 10
I explain to the student who just noticed
that diction, phrasing, and body language are choices

everyone makes, including someone
who looks like a shopping spree at *Flesh Crawls Tattoos.*
Egregious? I ask the room.

Standing out from the flock, a black sheep
the Greek chorus of a student answers.
You're not supposed to smile with a 10.

By definition, you're writhing.
Our patient writhes his gouty big toe
and the snake tattooed around his ankle.

He quotes me on why it's harder and harder to be a biped,
why it's easier and easier to blame gravity.
What I like about gout is Samuel Johnson had some too.

It's what a diet rich in DNA might do.
What I like about gout is the dietary history.
Who these days still fries a kidney for breakfast?

What is baloney full of?
What I like about gout is how uric acid
is handled in the hypertensive kidney,

how every kidney is smarter than its owner,
how lead in the wine jar gave the ancient Greeks gout,
why if it's not a nice Latinate word

chances are it's a nice Greek word,
why looking back it's still hard to believe
that what happened at that toga party

actually stayed there.
Don't do anything dumb on Facebook
I remind the innocent student.

What I don't like about gout is how *Pharma* cornered the market.
What I like about gout is how it comes and goes and comes and goes.
But chronic pain—the thing without feathers—

spends most of its life on the sofa.
It's also the thing without Medicaid
until the disability judge rules in its favor.

It interferes with activities of daily living
except for computer games that bleep
while blasting aliens into the bytes they came from.

That's not exactly constructive use of leisure time,
but it beats worrying about phantom pain in places
where even the urologist can't go.

When I diagram the gate theory of pain
and use the broken thermostat analogy
to point out a series of ascending opportunities

where non-opioid meds down regulate sensory pathways
and make it a little easier to live,
our patient smiles the way students in the back-row smile

when I derive the equation that converts common sense
into Bayesian gobbledygook.
We're somewhere between anger and pity

when I write the prescription he had to beg for.
He tries and tries but he can't teach me anything.
Hapless doctors are each hapless in different ways.

That's when I need Sadie—the generic non-shedding therapy dog—
to stroll into clinic in her cute little *working dog* vest
smelling all lavender and hypoallergenic.

My shoe passes her sniff test.
If dogs can sense the early treatable stage of lung cancer,
low blood sugar about to get ugly,

conception by day seven, a seizure on the way
or other non-ticking human bombs,
then they can sense who in the room

has *Milk Bones* in his pocket. *Sit* I command.
Sadie looks me in the eye, but I don't make her beg.
How do we salvage our sinking hearts I ask the flickering ceiling.

The fluorescent light is on the yellow side of white,
and everyone looks a little jaundiced.
The students may not carry dog treats, but they are smarter and smarter,

and every once in a while they need a rhetorical question
to chew on. We train them to measure everything
and when they get to the immeasurable they look down, look up, look back,

and change the subject to vertigo.
Socrates reminded his students that every case of gout is sickness
but all sickness isn't gout. Skipping ahead half a page

his logic gets to foolishness and tyranny.
No one wants to get in an argument with Socrates,
and maybe his reasoning made more sense

when light was slow and the sun orbited the earth
and the atomic nature of earth, air, fire, and water was barely a metaphor.
It's either easier or harder than it looks to be Socratic.

Leading the discussion from one false dichotomy to the next
often leads to getting another CT scan just to be sure
we're not missing something.

How do we account for uncertainty? I ask the student
who chances are hasn't flipped a coin
10 times then 20 times then 100 times

to learn how misleading either/or can be.
To predict the worst day of someone's life
will be better the day after

depends on chance getting the job done
during a steady state in an unbiased system
and the patience to wait till tomorrow.

When the day after the day after
the smart money strolls in for a check-up
and after the last act of the complete exam,

humility restored, one foot in the air looking for the empty leg,
that's when I remind myself that rich or poor
being a biped is no walk in the park.

If some of us are more human than others,
more ticklish for instance,
would Socrates then ask if some of us are less?

Or all of us are both, and some days more than others?
Forget Socrates, the student wants to know
if he heard what I heard when he listened to the heart.

Hearts don't speak, but they do murmur.
Students need feedback, and lunch,
but first we sit down, take a deep breath,

and take half a minute to pay close attention
to our own thumping tell-tale hearts.
Here it comes, there it goes. Here it comes.

At Medical Center Hour

a developmental biologist shows us a video of a fertilized egg
dividing into two then four then eight cells,
a day's worth of differentiation in a minute,
followed by a slide of a week old blastocyst drawn in cross section
with an outer cell mass or future placenta and an inner cell mass
that's either someone already or destined to be someone
with the same constitutional rights as any non-incarcerated citizen,
and while on the subject of genes as destiny the next clip
shows an unfertilized stem cell donated by a monkey at a lab
where the genetic basis of alcoholism is put to the test:
the stem cell donor sits in the corner of a cage, big smile on her face
since she was randomized to drink as much beer as her genes wanted,
and while that was supposed to be funny
it wasn't as funny as the story of the pope who decreed
that no human eggs could be stored in Italian laboratory freezers,
prompting wily Italian scientists to freeze dry eggs
for room air storage and quick and easy shipment to countries without popes,
but who needs eggs when stem cells on their own
can be encouraged to divide and divide and divide—virgin birth—
and keep dividing through the first trimester
at which point all they need to do is grow
until anyone who couldn't do *in vivo* or afford *in vitro* can have kids
which gives popes and Congress something else to think not very clearly about,
and something we don't really want to think about
is the electron micrograph of sperm speckled with HIV—
like ants at a picnic—
the price sperm pay for being sheltered from the immune system.
Thanks to enzymes like HIV's reverse transcriptase,
the human genome is at least 5% retroviral—
don't even try to parse which is which—
but those days when you don't feel altogether you?
We're all pink on the inside, and stained.

Like All Perfect Strangers

we'd have less trouble getting to the point
were it not for all the dogs wandering around
and the curious ways that *Middlemarch*

is everywhere. A few miles of George Eliot on audio
covers a lot of ground.
It doesn't take long to figure out

that Dorothea will need 600 pages
to let herself be happy. Attention spans are shorter now.
We'd met before, back when my classmates and I

were either right about everything
or worried about everything, and everything—
this was med school—smelled like formaldehyde.

Middlemarch was my idea of fun,
as if that kind of fun was the answer
to not knowing how to not study.

We'd take the whole brain out of the bucket
and put the pieces back.
Understanding the brain by thinking about it

is like understanding the lung by breathing hard
when biking to work and teaching dogs
they couldn't bark fast enough to catch me.

The dog labs didn't teach us anything
we couldn't have learned in a book,
but maybe dispassion in the name of science

was worth killing a few dogs for?
Like all eager students, we did what we were told,
and when we couldn't sleep we got up, opened a book,

and after reviewing a few neural pathways
pictured Dorothea biking to work like the rest of us.
She'd look righteous even in the spandex.

In chapter two George Eliot quotes Cervantes
with Quixote looking down the road seeing what he wants to see,
first in Spanish then in English.

By then we're coasting down the hill to clinic
where the non-English speaking Spanish patients
smile in defense. They've crossed the border to a strange land

where no one even attempts the subjunctive
and appointments get lost in translation.
Half way through explaining how hypertension

in the eye is not unlike hypertension in the kidney—
the same for diabetes—
it turns out *exudate* in Spanish is *exudate*,

or close enough. While he's at it, the interpreter—
there for back-up—undoes the double negatives.
Not that he's not right, but if the patient doesn't have

this, this, or this, then he couldn't have
that, that, or that, at least not very often.
I gave a paper once in Spanish.

The dean down there invited my dean
and my dean sent me. The early days of AIDS
and since no one knew what they were talking about

what I knew or how I said it hardly mattered.
There was a sidewalk on the seawall.
There was an ocean I was used to.

There was a fort that kept the English out.
Exudate: from the Latin for ooze,
as in looking out the window

where they're pouring concrete.
Those guys look like they speak Spanish.
¡Exudativo! they might exult,

calling and waving for more concrete.
Body Spanish sounds like body English.
In the audio section of the Advanced Spanish App

an American diplomat named Mr. White—
with the accent to prove it—is walking down the sidewalk
seeing what he wants to see, first in English

than in Spanish. There's the ocean he tells himself,
el mar for him, *la mer* were he a sailor.
He has crossed the border to a strange land

where words have genders and the rules
for masculine or feminine make exceptions.
The Molinas have invited him over for lunch.

They'll teach him how to say he's hungry,
how to say that's enough. More than enough
it might turn out. They're at the top of the hill

in a nice home behind a concrete wall
half again as tall as the police at every corner
of nice neighborhoods. Those police dogs

don't move or speak until they're told to.
The half-life of a policeman is shorter down there
than it is here. They get made examples of, but it's a job

and even a dangerous job is safer than none,
you'd hope. Besides, don't we all need the money
and count on luck?

After food and shelter money can't buy happiness.
Really? Depends on how you spend it.
If you're happy and you know it wag your tail

our dogs teach whenever they're done scratching.
Of course, they have food and shelter and all their shots.
When a patient brings a therapy dog to clinic—

dignity and purpose on a short leash—
our collective suffering and witnessing
will sit still, sit straight, stop whining and begging.

Dorothea has a dog named Monk and so do we.
She talks to Monk but George Eliot doesn't say what.
George Eliot doesn't say what when she doesn't have to.

Our Monk, a self-taught therapy dog,
rests his head in my lap when I'm typing.
At obedience school back in Miami during the drug wars

a drug dealer's dog bit ours. Drug dealer because
his dog would fly over a wall if told to,
and who else wears a Panama hat at night?

Those are loose criteria for diagnosing drug dealers,
and not all jerks are drug dealers, and not all dog owners
whose dog bites ours are jerks. In the county hospital ICU

where everybody went after getting shot
we made *¿que es mas macho? rounds,*
one desperado after another, each desperate

in his own way, each the victim of swift poetic justice.
Most of us spoke enough Spanish to know
what hurt or bled or leaked or even with hospital *Jell-O*

remained a little too unsettled.
Speaking of unsettled: if I were Mr. White I'd be mindful of
cerebriform chunks in the soup du jour.

Host families aren't kidding around when they serve that.
¿Pollo? I asked my *Doña* back in the steep days
of my learning curve. Mr. White might prefer the alphabet soup,

but either he doesn't know how to say that
or he's being diplomatic. Once we notice something
it's full of everything: grey matter, white matter,

whatever's the matter. Dr. Lydgate, the up-to-date
reductionist in *Middlemarch*, could reason his way
from soup to nuts, but he could only explain or question

or justify one thing at a time. That's true of all fiction.
Readers or listeners can look out the window
and get the big picture. We can go past outcome

to process, stop at a sidewalk too new to walk on
and wonder: wouldn't the concrete mixer,
a gyroscope at heart, resist turning a corner?

No matter how much you know about a gyroscope
or a bike or a gyroscope with pedals or a nerve
or the synapse where two nerves meet and braid

it won't help you make up your mind or discover
where you lost or found that train of thought.
The whole of you at any moment remains you,

greater than the sum of your parts regardless
how your day has been.
When our dogs take us for a walk after dinner

we notice what isn't something
that dogs have any business licking.
We notice the bats are still missing.

They should be fluttering past knowingly.
We hear the wood thrush whistle and thrash
and watch swallows dive and soar in flutterless arcs.

Flight is to swallows as exultation is to larks,
not that there are any larks around here.
Exultation is to happiness as one fluttering bat

is to knowing not to ask too much.
One fluttering bat is all.
Patients can't help it if they ask too much

when it seems like no one listens.
We're looking out the window or looking up
the Spanish word for elbow.

They're hoping *elbow* is the only thing
this *doctore* doesn't know.
My Spanish is good enough to dream in

but only in the present tense.

This Is Not a Drill

At work there are three kinds of drills: fire, earthquake, shooter.
During a fire drill the building empties into the parking lot
where crowds kill time and blame the fire marshal.
The smokers want to smoke but don't.
A doctor talks to the 2:40 patient and tries to stay on schedule.
If communication is the heart of medicine,
diligence is its habit. Then he looks for the 3:00 patient.

In a 5th floor office the photograph of a storm-tossed schooner
is ten degrees off plumb because that wasn't a drill.
Nor was it a backhoe unburying the storm drain it buried last month.
The walls shook while everyone wondered around looking for direction.
The Director said *this isn't my fault.* Then the world returned to normal.

As instructed: people keep quiet during the shooter drill.
They stare at the floor. They don't share funny looks.
Not only is it bad luck to reveal where you'd hide, it's unthinkable.
But if you look out the window and take a fire-escape moment
to consider all your options, you have to admit—
the inescapable fact of existence—
there's no corner small enough, no air thin enough, to disappear in.

Upstairs, when housekeeping straightens the photograph,
the Director restores the commemorative tilt.
The photographer spoke seven languages
and in a Tower of Babel accent recalled the wars he escaped
and the evil he didn't. Meanwhile, that ship is beached.
That sky is gray, that tide is lost, that storm is spent,
those sails are torn and empty.

The poet's recurrent dream is a sailboat that floats on air
and travels in time. He tacks back and forth over the old neighborhood
where old friends are still young. They look up, smile,
wave hello—goodbye—see you later. He'd wave back,
but one hand for the tiller, one hand for the sheet.
Even in a dream it's easy to spill the wind.
Even in a dream it takes practice.

Sleep Hygiene

Outline the night and all its objects in black magic marker.

The world through closed eyes needs texture
the way tires need tread,
brains need wrinkles, and hypnosis
needs the power of suggestion.
Traction, surface area, and control
might also apply to a cat
buried alive underneath the sheets:
if so, don't forget the one on top.

Stay up for several nights before
the night you plan to sleep.

Oil the ceiling fan.

True or false: the bladder
is on a separate circuit?

Don't eat in bed, especially chips.

Snoring + sleep apnea + restless legs
+ hemorrhoids + lumbago = the human condition.

The winter itch as well would be unfair.

Use pillows to solve or suppress all of the above,
a pillow shaped like the horizon
or the supine profile of your partner, or even better
a partner who won't mind being your pillow—

together you become the mountains and their clouds,
between the two of you a hidden canyon,
lost in your slopes there are deep limestone caves,
hot springs, the occasional tremor
of tectonic plates and knees.

Standing in Line at *Pet Forum*

while two girls were trying to decide how many crickets
for their lizard or whether it might save time, money, karma, and gas

to buy a plague of locusts,
I noticed the display of lasers for teasing cats.

It turns out that string works better for ours.
We've always had cats, and once a kitten-size reptile,

a Chinese water dragon with red eyes and cold blood
who taught us how it feels to be the object of indifference.

For years we had crickets on the shopping list,
but now I can put a red dot on anything I see,

or bounce it off the mirror where my wife's reflection
is removing earrings. I hoped to see her arch her back,

prepare to pounce, and pounce,
as if bringing home a field mouse.

But she refused the bait.
Later in bed with the lights off I traced

"I LOVE YOU" on the ceiling in foot tall letters,
but that kind of writing doesn't last.

She thought I was talking to myself again
or working something out or just playing with a streak of light

that jiggles at your pleasure.
She warned me not to shine it in anyone's eye—

her solar eclipse tone of voice—as if that would ever occur to me.
What happens is

you need people to notice what's dancing up their leg.

Bulkheads

There are dozens of ways to 360.
It's mostly in the hips

he promises.
We never know when

the ocean might surprise us.
What if an arm or two gets tangled up

in harpoon line?
What if suddenly

it's time to paddle upside down?
My leukemic friend and kayak mentor

is counting on remission, a year or more
including time

to teach me how to roll
like an Inuit.

Because of him I've added bulkheads
fore and aft, watertight,

silicon caulk, and lots of it.
He wants us to go out and play in the surf,

capsize for fun, for adventure,
for the sense of revival.

He can spin like a dolphin,
float like a cork, regulate

his angular momentum.
He knows when

to get nowhere fast and how
on a whim

to return to where he started.
There's no reason not to trust him.

In Memoriam

We shuffle into place and grieve in stanzas.
The acoustics cling like lint and everything—
family man, scholar, citizen, soldier—
sounds fuzzy and unraveled.
I read the hymns on my neighbor's lips.
I count the panes of stained glass.
The windows are too kind—
saints in post-beatitude poses
as if their share of suffering
is over, blame placed, sins forgiven,
and all they have to do now
is exemplify faith and endurance
the way models in catalogues
smile at the sea and stay young.
The sky is too blue, robes too soft,
martyrdom too therapeutic.
I explore my dark suit's pockets—
a prescription pad, a photo ID,
a list of people who expect a call,
a list of errands (birdseed, fertilizer),
a list of wards and numbered diagnoses.
Afterwards, there's a reception up the hill
but I am chiming like a clock
and rush off after letting the survivors
one at a time thank me for everything.

Swimming with John's Ghost

During the service, after the *mensch* acclamation
and before the sermon-sized metaphor
that started with a tree then lost me,
a comrade from the morning shift at college—
they shared a lecture hall and the appreciation
that all sleepy students are each sleepy in different ways—
quoted John bragging about having the North Grounds pool
all to himself at sunrise. Morning people brag
about their mornings. This morning the lifeguards,

proving they do pay attention to the lives they guard,
have the music tuned to oldies—Sam Cooke crooning
you-ou-ou-ou send me as Sam's fans adjust their goggles.
John, easy to spot in that deep blue bathing cap
he claims helps part the waters, takes the lane next to me.
We're standing there praying the water isn't as cold as it is
and waiting for one of us to acknowledge our existence.
Bummer about that service I say, hoping not to sound
too relieved he doesn't want to share my lane.
Total he says. Then we submerge. Strange how dying
helped his stroke. He doesn't have to breathe but does—
old habits die hard.

I'm a little choked up in the locker room
and he suggests *doing something about that cough.*
He would know. Since it is a locker room
I share some locker room wisdom:
when the going gets tough the tough get going.
John takes his cue: *practice doesn't make perfect,*
perfect practice makes perfect. We allow a moment of silence,
but before any hymns erupt I share my favorite hymn fact:
Emily Dickinson poems can be sung to the tune of *Amazing Grace.*
I dwell in pos-si-bil-i-ty he sings almost on key,
then asks if he can borrow my brush. *Get real* I answer.
Who wants to catch someone else's static?
We complain about chlorine and dry itchy skin.
We put our pants on one leg at a time,
an act of faith that grounds us. *See you later* he promises
and just like anyone walks out the door.

Last Day

It's my job to empty a plastic bag
filled with meds both past and present
and read out loud the labels of those we stopped,

and explain why, and while we're on why
why he needs oxygen at night, and the rescue inhaler.
Between pills it's my job to ask in a generic way

about life outside the clinic? He takes out his phone
because his story needs a prop.
His ex called yesterday, *only one ex, one's enough,*

just kids then, just friends now,
and she goes on and on, what if what if what if,
but after a while he has to do his business and promises to call back,

but forgets until something suddenly reminds him to call.
A half second later, half the speed of premonition,
his phone rings and rings and rings—her sister, a niece, a cousin—

and not just to chat. Silence needs a moment to sink in.
He snaps his fingers. *Just like that* is how.
He shrugs. *Out of the blue* in case I wondered.

He shows me the phone one more time to make sure,
then goes back to building a tower of bottles to take home.
I build a tower that stays here.

I always owe someone a call.
Maybe my job owes him a condolence note, or something?
He may not remember, or decided to forget,

today's my last day.
We give that a moment too.
He takes a long hit from his puffer.

He looks at me then through me, then a wheeze, then a sigh.
You're my boy he exhales,
and that's it for goodbye.

Even After Retiring

I read the obits and recognize patient names
and visit a website to sign a virtual guest list
that invites me to add a comment

after proving twice I'm not a bot.
It's harder than it looks to be real and earn permission
to greet the daughters and sons who helped me understand

that their mom drove everyone half nuts,
that the secret to her power
was never ever throwing a newspaper away

while feeding every stray cat who showed up on her porch.
It took her a while to teach me that her prior doctor,
a saint, with miracles and martyrdom to prove it,

did it his way, and just because that made no sense to me
didn't mean it might not work for her.
May she rest in peace.

May her family get some well-earned rest.
May that stuffed and lonely house find a seller's market.
May those strays find barns and live happy ever after.

May doctors not be saints. May saints not be martyrs.
May it be noted and recorded that she was lavish in praise
each time we scrolled through the cats on my phone.

Advance Directives

And should I ever appear in shorts that need suspenders
because my hips and butt have slid under the glacier of old age,
you are directed to suspend all life support measures including,
but not limited to, a glazed Krispy Kreme and a fountain Coca-Cola for lunch
because the lunch I packed got left behind on the kitchen counter
(not the first time this week to think ahead and make a lunch
and then rushing out the door forget I thought ahead)
and the donut was just sitting there—like plums in the Williams poem—
behind the nurse's desk at the clinic.
If I can't reach out and put the Slurpee straw between my lips
and slurp away while driving from hospital to house call, please don't do that for me, and
while you are not doing that you may as well stay off the subject of driving.
When you think about all the morons on the road
my habit of hugging the right curb is not as pathetic as it may seem to our kids,
who, like all kids, have short memories re: failure to yield or put gas in the tank.

I tell patients there are three things that get better with age:
emotional intelligence (staying calm under fire), resistance to the common cold,
and I can't remember the third...just kidding: scars.
The old ones are hidden by wrinkles and the new ones fade away
like fog or short-term memory.

Going back to the shorts: if lederhosen, don't wait for nature to strip me bare.

I'd like a non-denominational service that includes chariots but excludes flames.
Not even sparklers. I like the song "Take me Jesus, take me, take me to the Promised Land"
because that sounds like fun even though I don't believe in either and my faith,
coming out of the Borscht tradition, is barely an old wound that itches on the Sabbath.

If my heart stops or my breathing quits, recall that I'm a private person
who likes some peace and quiet and the key to the safe deposit box is in the copper bowl.

You know those boxers with pictures of sailboats? Dinghies to tall ships?
Ship me out in those.

To put my ashes in the garden as we discussed now strikes me as sicker
than fertilizing with night soil. I'm ok with the coffee can in the trunk of the car,
like my friend's uncle, or the sweater drawer with my father.
Temporarily of course, in anything, then anywhere, underneath the burning bush.
An urn would be too earnest.

Christmas Bird Count

Once upon a time in a century long ago
on the grounds of a proud university
built a century before that,

a dean, sitting in judgment, suddenly stands
and rushes to a window where
the cedar waxwings have arrived!

As they do every year regardless
whose interview they interrupt.
When those things with feathers flittered by

I was hoping for the job I still have.
Today we're hoping for a winter wren.
We're a few days short of winter, but there's snow.

There's a cedar waxwing in a cedar.
There are bluebirds wherever we need them.
That's not just a sparrow but a fox sparrow.

I look at my wife. She looks at me.
You call that a sparrow?
Maybe not. Or maybe yes.

I trust the guy with the serious optics.
It's easy to see why this farm is famous for its views
and dirt. That's not just bark, that's mulch.

Those aren't just leaves, that's compost.
Good dirt takes time. Views need distance.
That ridge is blue when the right cloud floats by.

This is fun an inner voice reminds. It's also cold.
Eyes and ears are learning something new.
Toes are not so interested, nor fingers,

but they're good sports.
The experts look warm. Thus expertise.
Between birds they compare hand warmers,

and one thing I've learned today is not to come back
without one of those rechargeable gizmos
in each pocket. It's Sunday morning, and the winter wren

is church enough for me. It looks like a wren
and sings like an angel. The Christmas bird count,
or *CBC* in the invitation,

is a week and a day before Christmas,
and one hundred years old today.
There used to be enough birds that birders shot

as many as it took to be merry.
In my day job CBC is complete blood count.
Some days my day job lasts all night.

If we still had to count the cells ourselves
no one could miss seeing
a bone marrow starting to be in a hurry.

My young colleague thinks a mistake is against the rules.
If so, Moses did not list it.
While waiting for grace or the Old Testament equivalent

is the perfect time to reappraise
the brightest stars in the visible heavens.
Looking up in wonder doesn't make us any warmer.

We shrug into a deeper layer.
I remind him I've made all his mistakes plus mine.
I remind him we'll be perfect again in the morning.

He asks if I heard the winter's tale
about the old guy in a long coat
who flashes across the subway track

where an old lady takes a long look before opining
you call that a lining? Yes, I'd heard.
Yes, I was ready to change the subject.

He heard it from his dad, I heard it from mine.
Thus diaspora.
He points to where Orion's nebula should be.

Or maybe not. Or maybe yes.
We shrug deeper in our deepest layer.
My coat, cozy as a thermos, as a paradox,

has a silver lining that reflects the cold
and absorbs the warmth us warmbloods need.
I need the boot equivalent of that coat,

boots that stay warm while slushing around
praying for the winter wren.
So after the CBC I go to the new shopping center

our city is so proud of and didn't need.
Ten thousand years from now hominids
will look at a mound on a ridge, take out their trowels,

uncover *Dick's Sporting Goods* and *Field and Stream*—
the retail equivalent of fraternal twins—
and theorize—in a Monday morning quarterbacking kind of way—

about afterlives and fantasy lives and inner lives
of a civilization that kills for sport, plays tackle football,
and reveres camo. Meanwhile, back at the ranch,

beyond the cross-bow aisle, past rifles in all calibers,
next to a statue of rutting deer, under a wall-size handgun sign—
we are an open carry state—

there's an aisle of boots in all sizes and seasons.
There's a mob of happy shoppers.
They aren't Chanukah shoppers.

Since the Nazis marched into town last August
I'm prone to that Jew at the Country Club feeling.
Proud old *Gone with the Wind*-style plantations

make good country clubs and golf courses.
Golf courses make good bird habitat,
not that I play golf. Not that we light a Menorah back at our ranch.

The other pole of my bipolar disorder
is secular Jew seeking winter solstice solace
in the new *iMax* as the new *Star Wars* unreels.

Who doesn't revere that jump to hyperspace?
Who doesn't need a festival of light?
Our Christmas tree started off as a mother-in-law device—

the ornaments, especially the dangling birds and fish,
gave us something to talk about.
Maybe two Moby Dicks aren't enough?

Whales aren't fish? Reread the novel but this time
don't skip the Wikipediesque sections on natural history.
Speaking of whiteness and all it stands for:

some of the white folks around here have had their feelings hurt.
All the black folks around here have had more than feelings hurt.
My wife and I met in Boston and notice that people here

talk funny and live in the past.
That ridge, that there ridge, made it hard to plant plantations.
Hence the Louisiana Purchase.

Whence manifest destiny.
Thus history.
Our tree could use some Marx and Engel action figures

engaged in playful dialectical materialism.
Troubled times, and what helps a little
is when the sales clerk calls me *Sugar*.

I also answer to *Honey*.
What helps a little is to help decorate our tree,
to put the loyal blue bird at the top of the tree

and work our way down. In such moments
a happy marriage lives happy ever after.
It seems only yesterday since that first big date

on the first *First Night* in Boston, a cold cold night,
but young love was and is a furnace.
Just kids then, now our kids aren't even kids.

Despite all that's wrong in the world
it spins just the way we like it,
and there's time to bundle up and see, hear, name and marvel

at what has arrived on time and in tune.
In my day job I'm a professional optimist.
When I tell someone *no new bad news*

he says wonderful. When I say *one step at a time*
she donates the walker to *Good Will.*
When I can't complement those poor old diabetic feet

I complement the socks.
If you can't trust smart wool, what can you trust?
Cold hands warm heart applies to feet too.

Toes warmers make perfect stocking stuffers.
Hand warmers like to be held.
Being easy to please isn't easy.

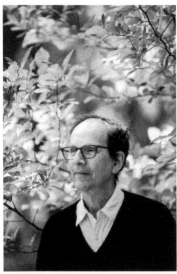

photo by Kristen Finn

Daniel Becker practiced and taught internal medicine at the University of Virginia School of Medicine until he retired in 2018. Now, he practices and teaches part-time and as a volunteer.

The New Issues Poetry Prize

Daniel M. Becker, *2nd Chance*
2019 Judge: Jericho Brown

Chet'la Sebree, *Mistress*
2018 Judge: Cathy Park Hong

Nina Puro, *Each Tree Could Hold a Noose or a House*
2017 Judge: David Rivard

Courtney Kampa, *Our Lady of Not Asking Why*
2016 Judge: Mary Szybist

Sawnie Morris, *Her, Infinite*
2015 Judge: Major Jackson

Abdul Ali, *Trouble Sleeping*
2014 Judge: Fanny Howe

Kerrin McCadden, *Landscape with Plywood Silhouettes*
2013 Judge: David St. John

Marni Ludgwig, *Pinwheel*
2012 Judge: Jean Valentine

Andrew Allport, *the body | of space | in the shape of the human*
2011 Judge: David Wojahn

Jeff Hoffman, *Journal of American Foreign Policy*
2010 Judge: Linda Gregerson